OSTEOPOROSIS DIET COOKBOOK FOR WOMEN OVER 60

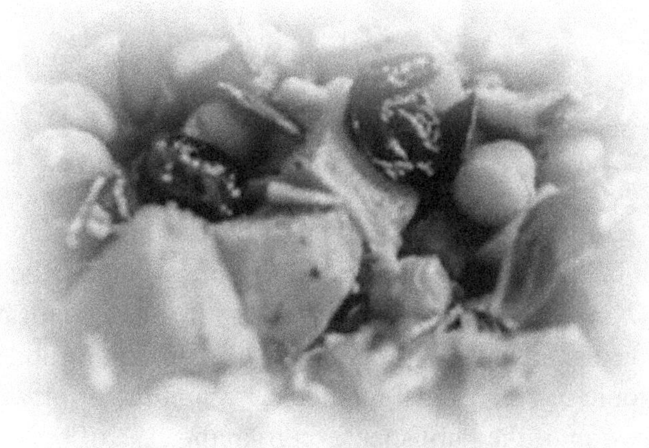

Healthy and Delicious Recipes to prevent, manage, and treat osteoporosis

David T. Salcedo

Copyright © 2023 by **David T. Salcedo**

TABLE OF CONTENTS

INTRODUCTION 7

WHAT IS OSTEOPOROSIS 9

   Causes of Osteoporosis 9

   Symptoms of Osteoporosis 10

   Treatment for Osteoporosis 11

   Preventive Measures 11

RISK FACTORS FOR WOMEN OVER THE AGE OF 60 12

NUTRITIONAL IMPORTANCE IN BONE HEALTH 17

DAILY CONSUMPTION OF THE LISTED NUTRIENTS 22

FOOD TO INCLUDE AND FOOD TO AVOID 26

   Food to Include 26

   Food to Avoid or Limit 28

CHAPTER 1 31

   Breakfast recipes 31

      1. Greek Yogurt with Berries and Almonds 31

      2. Spinach and Feta Omelet 32

      3. Quinoa Breakfast Bowl 33

      4. Whole Grain Pancakes with Nut Butter 34

      5. Berry Blast Smoothie 35

      6. Avocado Toast with Smoked Salmon 36

      7. Chia Seed Pudding with Mango 37

      8. Banana Nut Oatmeal 38

      9. Fruit and Nut Breakfast Quinoa Bowl 39

      10. Cottage Cheese and Pineapple Parfait 40

CHAPTER 2 41

Lunch recipes 41

1. Salmon and Quinoa Salad 41

2. Vegetable Stir-Fry with Tofu 42

3. Chicken and Spinach Whole Wheat Wrap 43

4. Mushroom and Spinach Quiche 44

5. Vegetarian Lentil Soup 45

6. Quinoa and Chickpea Salad.. 46

7. Sweet Potato and Kale Buddha Bowl........................... 47

8. Turkey and Veggie Wrap 48

9. Broccoli and Cheese Stuffed Baked Potatoes................ 49

10. Salad Niçoise with Grilled Tuna................................. 50

CHAPTER 3 51

Dinner recipes.. 51

1. Grilled Salmon with Lemon-Dill Sauce 51

2. Vegetarian Spinach and Chickpea Curry 52

3. Baked Chicken with Sweet Potato Mash....................... 53

4. Vegetable and Quinoa Stuffed Bell Peppers 54

5. Turkey and Vegetable Stir-Fry..................................... 55

6. Quinoa and Lentil Pilaf 56

7. Grilled Vegetable and Tofu Kebabs 57

8. Salmon and Asparagus Foil Packets............................. 58

9. Mushroom and Spinach Stuffed Chicken Breast........... 59

10. Quinoa and Kale Salad with Lemon-Tahini Dressing . 60

CHAPTER 4 61

Snacks Recipes 61

   1. Yogurt and Berry Parfait 61

   2. Cheese and Whole Grain Crackers 62

   3. Carrot and Hummus Dip 62

   4. Trail Mix with Nuts and Seeds 63

   5. Cottage Cheese with Pineapple 64

   6. Greek Yogurt and Almond Butter Dip 65

   7. Kale Chips 65

   8. Chia Seed Pudding with Berries 66

   9. Stuffed Celery with Cream Cheese 67

   10. Whole Grain Toast with Avocado 67

CHAPTER 5 69

Smoothies Recipes 69

   1. Berry Bliss Smoothie 69

   2. Green Goddess Smoothie 70

   3. Mango Tango Smoothie 71

   4. Banana Almond Delight 72

   5. Strawberry Kiwi Cooler 73

   6. Pineapple Mint Refresh 74

   8. Tropical Turmeric Smoothie 76

   9. Blueberry Spinach Power Smoothie 77

   10. Coconut Banana Dream 78

CHAPTER 6 79

7 days meal plan 79

   Day 1 79

Day 2 79

Day 3 79

Day 4 80

Day 5 80

Day 6 80

Day 7 80

CHAPTER 7 82

CONCLUSION 82

INTRODUCTION

I discovered a strong foe in the quiet corners of my life, where whispers of knowledge and echoes of experience reside, the understanding that my bones needed more treatment dawned on me as a woman over 60, like a gradual dawning. It wasn't simply a diagnosis; it was an invitation to go on a journey toward stronger, more robust bones.

This journey was about more than just fighting a disease; it was about self-discovery, resilience, and wonderful transformation via the power of food. In the pages that follow, I welcome you to accompany me on this journey, where every meal became a ritual of sustenance and every recipe a step toward regaining my skeletal strength.

As I descended into the maze of osteoporosis, I learned that the way to stronger bones was not a sterile prescription or a set of strict guidelines. On my kitchen counter, a culinary journey, a gastronomic odyssey unfolded. I could feel the rebirth of vitality within me with each carefully chosen ingredient and beautifully constructed dish.

This cookbook is more than just a dish collection; it's a story of resilience and joy, a celebration of the transformation that a well-balanced, bone-nourishing diet can bring. More than just culinary advice awaits you in the next chapters; you'll discover a road map to a life where every food is a step toward renewed health and well-being.

This book is an invitation to relish the journey, whether you're currently on a quest for bone health or just starting to think about the demands of your aging bones. It's a guarantee that the kitchen may be your haven, and that each meal can be a confession of love for your bones. Let's flip the page together, and may this book be your companion on your way to a life of stronger, more resilient bones.

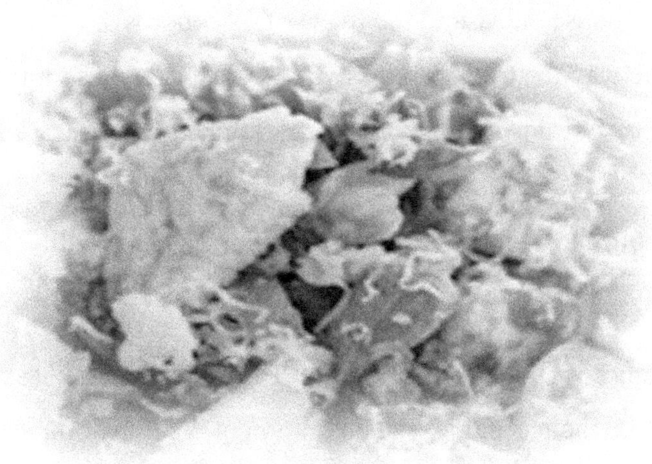

WHAT IS OSTEOPOROSIS

Osteoporosis is a disorder that gradually weakens bones, making them fragile and prone to fractures. This pernicious disease affects millions of people, primarily women over the age of 60. Understanding the reasons, detecting symptoms, researching treatment options, and implementing preventive measures are all critical aspects in the fight against osteoporosis.

Causes of Osteoporosis

Aging: As we get older, the natural process of bone remodeling slows down, resulting in a gradual decrease of bone density.

Changes in Hormones: Postmenopausal women undergo a considerable drop in estrogen, a hormone essential for bone density maintenance. This hormonal change contributes to faster bone loss.

Nutritional Deficiencies: A lack of calcium and vitamin D might jeopardize bone health. These nutrients are critical in maintaining bone strength and density.

Genetics: The chance of getting osteoporosis can be influenced by family history. A genetic proclivity for low bone density may enhance the risk.

Sedentary lifestyles, heavy alcohol intake, smoking, and a lack of weight-bearing activity are all risk factors for osteoporosis.

Symptoms of Osteoporosis

Fractures: Fragile bones are more prone to fractures, particularly in the hip, spine, and wrist. These fractures can occur with little or no impact.

Compression fractures in the spine can cause a gradual decrease of height over time.

Back Pain: Spinal fractures can produce chronic back pain, which is a common symptom of osteoporosis.

Treatment for Osteoporosis

Prescription drugs such as bisphosphonates, hormone treatment, and denosumab can help delay bone loss and lower the risk of fractures.

Calcium and vitamin D supplements: Adequate calcium and vitamin D intake is critical for bone health. Supplements may be advised, particularly if dietary intake is inadequate.

Weight-bearing workouts, such as walking or strength training, can help enhance bone density. Quitting smoking and limiting alcohol use also help with bone health.

Preventive Measures

Balanced Diet: Consume calcium and vitamin D-rich foods such as dairy products, leafy greens, and fortified meals.

Regular Exercise: To enhance bone strength, engage in weight-bearing exercises such as walking, running, or resistance training.

To lower the risk of bone loss, adopt a healthy lifestyle that includes quitting smoking and limiting alcohol consumption.

Regular bone density scans can help detect early signs of bone loss, allowing for appropriate intervention.

RISK FACTORS FOR WOMEN OVER THE AGE OF 60

Osteoporosis, a disorder characterized by weakening and porous bones, is a major health problem, especially among women over the age of 60. As women reach their forties, they encounter a confluence of circumstances that lead to an increased risk of osteoporosis. Understanding these risk factors is critical for the early discovery, prevention, and effective therapy of this bone disease.

Changes During Menopause

- Estrogen Decline: The hormonal changes associated with menopause, notably the decrease in estrogen levels, play a critical role in the development of osteoporosis. Estrogen is essential for bone density maintenance, and its decline after menopause hastens bone loss.

Bone Loss with Age

- Natural Bone Remodeling: The process of bone remodeling becomes less efficient as women age. The equilibrium between bone creation and resorption alters, resulting in gradual bone density loss.

History of the Family

- Genetic Predisposition: Having a family history of osteoporosis raises the chances of having the illness. Genetic factors can alter bone density and fracture propensity.

Deficiencies in Nutrition

- Calcium and Vitamin D Deficiency: A lack of calcium and vitamin D, both of which are necessary for bone health, can contribute to bone loss. Women's nutritional needs may rise as they age, and inadequacies become increasingly common.

Low Body Mass Index

- Underweight or petite Frame: Women who are underweight or have a petite frame have less bone mass to begin with, leaving them more vulnerable to osteoporosis and rapid bone loss.

Inactive Way of Life

- Lack of Weight-Bearing Exercise: Physical inactivity, particularly a lack of weight-bearing exercises such as walking, running, or resistance training, hastens bone loss and weakens bones over time.

Smoking

- Smoking is linked to reduced bone density and an increased risk of fractures. It also interferes with calcium absorption, putting bone health at risk.

Drinking Too Much Alcohol

- Alcoholism: Chronic and excessive alcohol intake can impair the body's ability to absorb calcium, contributing to bone density loss.

Medical Problems

- Hormonal diseases: Hyperthyroidism and adrenal diseases can both impact hormone levels and contribute to bone loss.
- Gastrointestinal Disorders: Conditions such as celiac disease and inflammatory bowel disease can impair nutrient absorption, resulting in deficits that harm bone health.

Medications

- Long-Term Use of Certain drugs: Certain drugs, such as corticosteroids and certain anti-seizure medications, might weaken bones if taken over a lengthy period of time.

Previous Breaks

- Fracture History: Women who have had previous fractures may be at a higher risk of future fractures, indicating underlying bone health concerns.

Ethnicity and race

- Asian and Caucasian Women: Asian and Caucasian women are at a higher risk of osteoporosis than women of other ethnic backgrounds.

Factors of Socioeconomic Status

- Limited Access to Healthcare: Socioeconomic issues that limit access to healthcare, particularly frequent check-ups and preventive screenings, can contribute to osteoporosis that goes unnoticed and untreated.

NUTRITIONAL IMPORTANCE IN BONE HEALTH

Bones, our bodies' quiet scaffolding, are not static structures but dynamic, living tissues that are continually rebuilding. Proper diet is essential for preserving bone strength and density throughout life. Understanding the role of nutrition in bone health is critical for preventing disorders such as osteoporosis and maintaining general health.

Calcium

- Calcium Absorption and Storage: Calcium is a fundamental mineral component of bones that provides structural integrity and strength. Calcium is essential for bone production, and the body stores it in the bones for later use.
- Calcium-Rich Foods: Dairy products, leafy greens, nuts, seeds, and fortified foods are high in calcium.

Vitamin D

- Calcium Absorption Enhancer: Vitamin D is essential for the body's proper absorption of calcium from the digestive tract.

- Sun Exposure and Dietary Sources: While sunshine is a natural source of vitamin D, fatty fish, egg yolks, and fortified foods are dietary sources that help to keep levels stable.

Vitamin K

- Bone Mineralization Support: Vitamin K is required for proper bone mineralization, which ensures that calcium is deposited in the bone matrix.

- Leafy Greens and Cruciferous Vegetables: Vitamin K-rich foods include kale, spinach, broccoli, and Brussels sprouts.

Magnesium

- Bone Structure: Magnesium helps to maintain bone structure and is involved in the conversion of vitamin D into its active form for calcium absorption.
- Nuts, Seeds, and Whole Grains: Foods high in magnesium include almonds, sunflower seeds, and whole grains.

Phosphorus

- Calcium Synergy: Phosphorus works in tandem with calcium to promote bone and tooth mineralization.
- Protein-Rich Foods: Phosphorus-containing foods include meat, dairy, and legumes.

Protein

- Structural Component: Protein is a crucial building ingredient of bone tissue that serves as a matrix for mineral deposition.
- Lean Meats, Beans, and Dairy: Eating lean meats, beans, and dairy products promotes enough protein intake for bone health.

Fruits and vegetables

- Anti-Inflammatory Properties: Antioxidants found in fruits and vegetables aid to reduce inflammation, thereby improving general bone health.
- Alkalizing impact: Some fruits and vegetables have an alkalizing impact, which may assist bone health by maintaining an ideal pH balance.

Omega-3 Fatty Acids

- Anti-Inflammatory Role: Omega-3 fatty acids, which can be found in fatty fish and flaxseeds, have anti-inflammatory characteristics that may help to prevent bone resorption.
- Maintaining a Balance of Omega-3 and Omega-6 Fatty Acids: Maintaining a balance of omega-3 and omega-6 fatty acids is critical for general bone health.

Keeping Bone-Depleting Factors to a Minimum

- Caffeine and Alcohol Moderation: Too much caffeine and alcohol can interfere with calcium absorption, thus moderation is essential.
- Be Aware of Your Salt consumption: A high salt consumption might cause increased calcium excretion in the urine, potentially affecting bone health.

DAILY CONSUMPTION OF THE LISTED NUTRIENTS

Calcium

Daily Value: 1,200-1,500 mg

Keep in mind that adequate calcium consumption is critical for bone health, especially in postmenopausal women.

Vitamin D

Recommended daily allowance: 600-800 IU

For optimal vitamin D levels, both sunlight exposure and food sources are considered.

Vitamin K

Daily Value: 90-120 mcg

Vitamin K promotes bone health by assisting in bone mineralization.

Magnesium

Daily Value: 320 mg

Magnesium is required for bone structure and calcium metabolism.

Phosphorus

Daily Value: 700 mg

Works with calcium to help in bone mineralization.

Protein

Daily Value: 46-56 grams

Protein is essential for bone tissue maintenance and overall wellness.

Omega-3 Fatty Acids

Daily Allowance (EPA and DHA combined): 1.1-1.6 g

Omega-3 fatty acids, found in fatty fish, flaxseeds, and walnuts, may help with bone health.

Vitamin C

Daily Value: 75 mg

Promotes collagen production, which is necessary for bone structure.

Vitamin A

Daily Value: 700-900 mcg

Required for bone formation and remodeling.

Zinc

Daily Value 8 mg

Aids in the mineralization and turnover of bones.

Copper

Daily Allowance: 900 mcg

Aids in the synthesis of collagen in the bones.

Vitamin (B6, B12, Folate)

Daily Allowance: B6: 1.5 mg, B12: 2.4 mcg and Folate: 400 mg

Participates in homocysteine metabolism and is connected to bone health.

Potassium

Daily Allowance: 2,600-3,100 mg

May aid in bone mineral density maintenance.

Selenium

Daily Allowance: 55 mcg

Antioxidant effects, maybe beneficial to bone health.

FOOD TO INCLUDE AND FOOD TO AVOID

Food to Include

Foods Rich in Calcium

Dairy products (low-fat or fat-free milk, yogurt, cheese), leafy greens (kale, broccoli), almonds, fortified plant-based milk (soy, almond) are good sources.

Vitamin D

Fatty fish (salmon, mackerel), egg yolks, fortified meals (orange juice, cereals) are good sources.

Leafy Greens

Sources: Calcium and other nutrients are abundant in spinach, kale, collard greens, and other dark, leafy vegetables.

Fruits and Vegetables

Sources: A wide range of fruits and vegetables include important vitamins, minerals, and antioxidants. Choose a bright arrangement.

Lean Protein

Protein sources include skinless poultry, fish, lean meats, beans, lentils, and tofu, which are low in saturated fat.

Omega-3 Fatty Acids

Fatty fish (salmon, sardines), flaxseeds, chia seeds, and walnuts are good sources.

Whole Grain

Sources: Magnesium and phosphorus are found in whole grain bread, brown rice, quinoa, oats, and whole wheat pasta.

Low-Fat Dairy

Sources: To limit saturated fat intake, choose low-fat or fat-free milk, yogurt, and cheese.

Nut and Seeds

Sources: Calcium, magnesium, and other nutrients can be found in almonds, sunflower seeds, chia seeds, and sesame seeds.

Herbs and Spices

Use anti-inflammatory herbs and spices such as turmeric, oregano, and basil.

Food to Avoid or Limit

High Sodium Foods

Processed foods, canned soups, and salty snacks are among examples.

Reason: Too much sodium might cause calcium excretion in the urine.

Excess Caffeine

Examples include coffee, tea, and caffeinated sodas.

Reason: Caffeine use may interfere with calcium absorption.

Alcohol

Restrict alcohol consumption.

The reason is that excessive alcohol use might interfere with calcium absorption and contribute to bone loss.

Foods High in Phosphorus

Some examples are colas, processed meats, and convenience foods.

Reason: Too much phosphorus can interfere with calcium absorption.

Foods High in Sugar

Sugary snacks, candy, and desserts are examples.

Reason: Sugary diets may contribute to inflammation and have a bad influence on bone health.

Foods that have been fried or processed

Examples include fast food and packaged snacks.

The reason is that it is high in harmful fats and may contribute to inflammation.

Certain Acidic Foods

Citrus fruits, tomatoes, and vinegar are some examples.

Reason: Consuming high-acid meals in excess may contribute to calcium loss.

Saturated Fats

Examples include fatty cuts of beef and full-fat dairy.

Reason: Saturated fat-rich diets may contribute to bone loss.

Excess Vitamin A

Sources include liver and high-dose supplements.

Reason: Excessive vitamin A consumption may have a harmful impact on bone health.

Deli Meats that have been processed

Examples include bacon, sausages, and deli meats.

Reason: High in salt and frequently containing preservatives that may be harmful to bone health.

CHAPTER 1

Breakfast recipes

1. Greek Yogurt with Berries and Almonds

Ingredients

- Greek yogurt

- Mixed berries (blueberries, strawberries)

- Almonds (sliced)

- Honey (optional)

Preparation

- Layer Greek yogurt with berries and sliced almonds in a glass.

- Drizzle with honey if desired.

Nutritional Information

- Protein-rich, high in calcium, vitamin C, and antioxidants.

Serving Size: 1 parfait

Preparation Time: 5 minutes

2. Spinach and Feta Omelet

Ingredients

- Eggs

- Fresh spinach

- Feta cheese (crumbled)

- Olive oil

Preparation

- Sauté spinach in olive oil until wilted.

- Whisk eggs and pour over spinach, add feta, cook until set.

Nutritional Information

- It is high in calcium, protein and vitamin k.

Serving Size: 1 omelet

Preparation Time: 10 minutes

3. Quinoa Breakfast Bowl

Ingredients

- Cooked quinoa

- Greek yogurt

- Mixed berries

- Chia seeds

Preparation

- Mix quinoa with Greek yogurt, top with berries and chia seeds.

Nutritional Information

- Excellent source of protein, fiber, and essential nutrients.

Serving Size: 1 bowl

Preparation Time: 15 minutes (if quinoa is pre-cooked)

4.Whole Grain Pancakes with Nut Butter

Ingredients

- Whole grain pancake mix

- Nut butter (almond, peanut)

- Banana slices

Preparation

- Prepare pancakes as per package instructions, spread with nut butter, and top with banana slices.

Nutritional Information

- Good source of whole grains, protein, and potassium.

Serving Size: 2-3 pancakes

Preparation Time: 15 minutes

5.Berry Blast Smoothie

Ingredients

- Mixed berries (strawberries, blueberries, raspberries)

- Greek yogurt

- Spinach

- Almond milk

Preparation

- Blend berries, yogurt, spinach, and almond milk until smooth.

Nutritional Information

- Packed with vitamins, minerals, and antioxidants.

Serving Size: 1 smoothie

Preparation Time: 5 minutes

6. Avocado Toast with Smoked Salmon

Ingredients

- Whole grain bread

- Avocado

- Smoked salmon

- Lemon juice

Preparation

- Mash avocado, spread on toast, top with smoked salmon, and a squeeze of lemon.

Nutritional Information

- It is good in omega-3 fatty acids, vitamin D, and fiber.

Serving Size: 1-2 slices

Preparation Time: 10 minutes

7. Chia Seed Pudding with Mango

Ingredients

- Chia seeds

- Almond milk

- Mango chunks

- Honey (optional)

Preparation

- Mix chia seeds with almond milk, refrigerate until pudding consistency, top with mango and honey.

Nutritional Information

- High in omega-3s, calcium, and vitamin C.

- **Serving Size:** 1 pudding

- **Preparation Time:** 5 minutes (plus refrigeration time)

8.Banana Nut Oatmeal

Ingredients

- Rolled oats

- Almond milk

- Banana slices

- Walnuts

Preparation

- Cook oats with almond milk, top with banana slices and crushed walnuts.

Nutritional Information

- It is highly nutritious in fiber, potassium, and omega-3 fatty acids.

Serving Size: 1 bowl

Preparation Time: 10 minutes

9. Fruit and Nut Breakfast Quinoa Bowl

Ingredients

- Cooked quinoa

- Mixed fruits (berries, kiwi, pineapple)

- Mixed nuts (almonds, walnuts)

Preparation

- Combine cooked quinoa with fruits and nuts.

Nutritional Information

- It is nutritious in protein, fiber, vitamins, and minerals.

Serving Size: 1 bowl

Preparation Time: 15 minutes (if quinoa is pre-cooked)

10. Cottage Cheese and Pineapple Parfait

Ingredients

- Low-fat cottage cheese
- Fresh pineapple chunks
- Granola

Preparation

- Layer cottage cheese with pineapple chunks and granola.

Nutritional Information

- It is nutritious in protein, calcium, and vitamin C.

Serving Size: 1 parfait

Preparation Time: 5 minutes

CHAPTER 2

Lunch recipes

1. Salmon and Quinoa Salad

Ingredients

- Grilled salmon fillet

- Cooked quinoa

- Mixed greens

- Cherry tomatoes

- Olive oil and lemon dressing

Preparation

- Combine quinoa, mixed greens, cherry tomatoes, and top with grilled salmon. Drizzle with olive oil and lemon dressing.

Nutritional Information

- It is nutritious in omega-3 fatty acids, protein, and calcium.

Serving Size: 1 plate

Preparation Time: 20 minutes

2. Vegetable Stir-Fry with Tofu

Ingredients

- Tofu cubes

- Assorted vegetables (broccoli, bell peppers, carrots)

- Brown rice

- Soy sauce

- Ginger and garlic

Preparation

- Stir-fry tofu and vegetables in soy sauce, garlic, and ginger. Serve over brown rice.

Nutritional Information

- High in plant-based protein, fiber, and essential nutrients.

Serving Size: 1 bowl

Preparation Time: 25 minutes

3.Chicken and Spinach Whole Wheat Wrap

Ingredients

- Grilled chicken strips

- Whole wheat wrap

- Fresh spinach leaves

- Hummus

- Cherry tomatoes

Preparation

- Spread hummus on the wrap, add grilled chicken, fresh spinach, and cherry tomatoes. Roll up and serve.

Nutritional Information

- Protein-packed with added calcium and vitamin K from spinach.

Serving Size: 1 wrap

Preparation Time: 15 minutes

4. Mushroom and Spinach Quiche

Ingredients

- Whole grain pie crust

- Eggs

- Mushrooms

- Fresh spinach

- Low-fat cheese

Preparation

- Whisk eggs, add sautéed mushrooms and spinach. Pour into pie crust, top with cheese, and bake.

Nutritional Information

- High in protein, calcium, and vitamin D.

Serving Size: 1 slice

Preparation Time: 30 minutes

5. Vegetarian Lentil Soup

Ingredients

- Lentils

- Mixed vegetables (carrots, celery, onions)

- Vegetable broth

- Spinach leaves

Preparation

- Cook lentils and vegetables in vegetable broth until tender. Add spinach before serving.

Nutritional Information

- High in fiber, plant-based protein, and essential vitamins.

Serving Size: 1 bowl

Preparation Time: 40 minutes

6. Quinoa and Chickpea Salad

Ingredients

- Cooked quinoa

- Chickpeas

- Cucumber

- Cherry tomatoes

- Feta cheese

Preparation

- Mix quinoa, chickpeas, cucumber, and cherry tomatoes. Top with crumbled feta.

Nutritional Information

- Excellent source of plant-based protein, calcium, and fiber.

Serving Size: 1 plate

Preparation Time: 15 minutes

7. Sweet Potato and Kale Buddha Bowl

Ingredients

- Roasted sweet potato cubes

- Kale (massaged with olive oil)

- Quinoa

- Avocado slices

- Tahini dressing

Preparation

- Assemble roasted sweet potatoes, massaged kale, quinoa, and avocado. Drizzle with tahini dressing.

Nutritional Information

- High in vitamin K, calcium, and essential nutrients.

Serving Size: 1 bowl

Preparation Time: 30 minutes

8. Turkey and Veggie Wrap

Ingredients

- Turkey slices

- Whole grain wrap

- Hummus

- Shredded carrots

- Spinach leaves

Preparation

- Spread hummus on the wrap, add turkey, shredded carrots, and spinach. Roll up and serve.

Nutritional Information

- Protein-rich with added vitamins and minerals from veggies.

Serving Size: 1 wrap

Preparation Time: 15 minutes

9. Broccoli and Cheese Stuffed Baked Potatoes

Ingredients

- Baked potatoes

- Steamed broccoli

- Low-fat cheese

- Greek yogurt (as a topping)

Preparation

- Scoop out the potato, mix with steamed broccoli, top with cheese, and bake. Add a dollop of Greek yogurt before serving.

Nutritional Information

- It is highly nutritious in calcium, vitamin C, and fiber.

Serving Size: 1 potato

Preparation Time: 40 minutes

10. Salad Niçoise with Grilled Tuna

Ingredients

- Grilled tuna steak
- Mixed greens
- Cherry tomatoes
- Hard-boiled eggs
- Kalamata olives

Preparation

- Assemble mixed greens, cherry tomatoes, hard-boiled eggs, and olives. Top with grilled tuna.

Nutritional Information

- Rich in omega-3s, protein, and various vitamins and minerals.

Serving Size: 1 plate

Preparation Time: 25 minutes

CHAPTER 3

Dinner recipes

1. Grilled Salmon with Lemon-Dill Sauce

Ingredients

- Salmon fillets
- Lemon juice
- Fresh dill
- Olive oil

Preparation

- Grill salmon, drizzle with a sauce made from lemon juice, fresh dill, and olive oil.

Nutritional Information

- High in omega-3 fatty acids, vitamin D, and calcium.

Serving Size: 1 fillet

Preparation Time: 20 minutes

2. Vegetarian Spinach and Chickpea Curry

Ingredients

- Chickpeas

- Spinach

- Tomatoes

- Coconut milk

- Curry spices

Preparation

- Cook chickpeas and spinach in a curry sauce made with tomatoes, coconut milk, and spices.

Nutritional Information

- Plant-based protein, fiber, and various vitamins and minerals.

Serving Size: 1 bowl

Preparation Time: 30 minutes

3. Baked Chicken with Sweet Potato Mash

Ingredients

- Chicken breasts

- Sweet potatoes

- Greek yogurt

- Garlic

Preparation

- Bake chicken and serve with mashed sweet potatoes mixed with Greek yogurt and garlic.

Nutritional Information

- High in protein, vitamin A, and potassium.

Serving Size: 1 serving

Preparation Time: 40 minutes

4. Vegetable and Quinoa Stuffed Bell Peppers

Ingredients

- Quinoa

- Bell peppers

- Mixed vegetables (zucchini, carrots, tomatoes)

- Feta cheese

Preparation

- Cook quinoa and mix with sautéed vegetables. Stuff bell peppers and bake. Top with feta.

Nutritional Information

- Protein-rich, high in fiber, and various vitamins.

Serving Size: 2 stuffed peppers

Preparation Time: 45 minutes

5. Turkey and Vegetable Stir-Fry

Ingredients

- Ground turkey

- Broccoli

- Snap peas

- Bell peppers

- Soy sauce

Preparation

- Stir-fry ground turkey with vegetables and soy sauce.

Nutritional Information

- Lean protein, fiber, and essential nutrients.

Serving Size: 1 plate

Preparation Time: 25 minutes

6. Quinoa and Lentil Pilaf

Ingredients

- Quinoa

- Lentils

- Onion

- Garlic

- Vegetable broth

Preparation

- Sauté onion and garlic, add quinoa, lentils, and vegetable broth. Simmer until cooked.

Nutritional Information

- Plant-based protein, fiber, and various vitamins and minerals.

Serving Size: 1 bowl

Preparation Time: 35 minutes

7. Grilled Vegetable and Tofu Kebabs

Ingredients

- Tofu cubes

- Bell peppers

- Zucchini

- Cherry tomatoes

- Balsamic glaze

Preparation

- Thread tofu and vegetables onto skewers, grill, and drizzle with balsamic glaze.

Nutritional Information

- Plant-based protein, vitamins, and antioxidants.

Serving Size: 1 skewer

Preparation Time: 30 minutes

8. Salmon and Asparagus Foil Packets

Ingredients

- Salmon fillets

- Asparagus spears

- Lemon slices

- Dill

Preparation

- Place salmon and asparagus on foil, season with lemon and dill, seal and bake.

Nutritional Information

- Rich in omega-3s, vitamin D, and antioxidants.

Serving Size: 1 packet

Preparation Time: 25 minutes

9. Mushroom and Spinach Stuffed Chicken Breast

Ingredients

- Chicken breasts

- Mushrooms

- Fresh spinach

- Low-fat cheese

Preparation

- Stuff chicken breasts with sautéed mushrooms, spinach, and cheese. Bake until cooked.

Nutritional Information

- It is nutritious in protein, calcium, and vitamin K.

Serving Size: 1 chicken breast

Preparation Time: 35 minutes

10. Quinoa and Kale Salad with Lemon-Tahini Dressing

Ingredients

- Cooked quinoa
- Kale leaves (massaged)
- Cherry tomatoes
- Avocado slices
- Lemon-tahini dressing

Preparation

- Combine quinoa, massaged kale, cherry tomatoes, and avocado.
- Drizzle with lemon-tahini dressing.

Nutritional Information

- High in plant-based protein, calcium, and essential nutrients.

Serving Size:1 bowl

Preparation Time:20 minutes

CHAPTER 4

Snacks Recipes

1. Yogurt and Berry Parfait

Ingredients

- Greek yogurt
- Mixed berries (blueberries, strawberries)
- Almonds (sliced)
- Honey (optional)

Preparation

- Layer Greek yogurt with berries and sliced almonds in a glass.
- Drizzle with honey if desired.

Nutritional Information

- High in calcium, vitamin D, antioxidants, and protein.

Serving Size: 1 parfait

Preparation Time: 5 minutes

2. Cheese and Whole Grain Crackers

Ingredients

- Whole grain crackers
- Cheese cubes (preferably high in calcium)

Preparation:

- Arrange whole grain crackers with cheese cubes.

Nutritional Information:

- Provides calcium and protein.

Serving Size: 1 serving

Preparation Time: 2 minutes

3. Carrot and Hummus Dip

Ingredients:

- Carrot sticks
- Hummus

Preparation:

- Dip carrot sticks into hummus.

Nutritional Information:

- High in vitamin A, fiber, and protein.

Serving Size: 1 serving

Preparation Time: 5 minutes

4. Trail Mix with Nuts and Seeds

Ingredients

- Almonds
- Walnuts
- Pumpkin seeds
- Sunflower seeds
- Dried fruits

Preparation

- Mix nuts and seeds with dried fruits to create a trail mix.

Nutritional Information

- Provides calcium, magnesium, and healthy fats.

Serving Size: 1 handful

Preparation Time: 2 minutes

5. Cottage Cheese with Pineapple

Ingredients

- Low-fat cottage cheese
- Fresh pineapple chunks

Preparation

- Cottage cheese should be combined with fresh pineapple chunks.

Nutritional Information

- It has high content of calcium, vitamin C, and protein.

Serving Size: 1 serving

Preparation Time: 3 minutes

6. Greek Yogurt and Almond Butter Dip

Ingredients

- Greek yogurt

- Almond butter

- Apple slices for dipping

Preparation

- Mix Greek yogurt with almond butter. Use apple slices for dipping.

Nutritional Information

- It is nutritious in calcium, protein, and healthy fats.

Serving Size: 1 serving

Preparation Time: 5 minutes

7. Kale Chips

Ingredients

- Fresh kale leaves

- Olive oil

- Sea salt

Preparation

- Coat kale leaves in olive oil, sprinkle with sea salt, and bake until crisp.

Nutritional Information

- It has high content in calcium, vitamin K, and antioxidants.

Serving Size: 1 bowl

Preparation Time: 15 minutes

8. Chia Seed Pudding with Berries

Ingredients

- Chia seeds

- Almond milk

- Mixed berries

Preparation

- Mix chia seeds with almond milk, refrigerate until pudding consistency, and top with mixed berries.

Nutritional Information

- Rich in omega-3s, calcium, and antioxidants.

Serving Size: 1 pudding

Preparation Time: 5 minutes (plus refrigeration time)

9. Stuffed Celery with Cream Cheese

Ingredients

- Celery sticks

- Low-fat cream cheese

Preparation

- Celery sticks should be filled with low-fat cream cheese.

Nutritional Information:

- Provides calcium and a crunch.

Serving Size: 1 serving

Preparation Time: 3 minutes

10. Whole Grain Toast with Avocado

Ingredients

- Whole grain bread
- Avocado
- Lemon juice

Preparation

- Mash avocado, spread on whole grain toast, and squeeze lemon juice on top.

Nutritional Information

- High in fiber, vitamin K, and healthy fats.

Serving Size:1-2 slices

Preparation Time: 5 minutes

CHAPTER 5

Smoothies Recipes

1. Berry Bliss Smoothie

Ingredients

- Mixed berries (strawberries, blueberries, raspberries)
- Greek yogurt
- Spinach leaves
- Almond milk

Preparation

- Blend berries, Greek yogurt, spinach, and almond milk until smooth.

Nutritional Information

- Rich in antioxidants, calcium, and vitamin K.

Serving Size: 1 smoothie

Preparation Time: 5 minutes

2. Green Goddess Smoothie

Ingredients

- Kale leaves

- Pineapple chunks

- Banana

- Chia seeds

- Coconut water

Preparation

- Blend kale, pineapple, banana, chia seeds, and coconut water until creamy.

Nutritional Information

- High in calcium, vitamin C, and omega-3 fatty acids.

Serving Size: 1 smoothie

Preparation Time: 7 minutes

3. Mango Tango Smoothie

Ingredients

- Mango chunks

- Low-fat yogurt

- Flaxseeds

- Orange juice

Preparation

- Blend mango, yogurt, flaxseeds, and orange juice until smooth.

Nutritional Information

- It is nutritious in vitamin D, calcium, and fiber.

Serving Size: 1 smoothie

Preparation Time: 5 minutes

4. Banana Almond Delight

Ingredients

- Banana

- Almond butter

- Spinach leaves

- Almond milk

Preparation

- Blend banana, almond butter, spinach, and almond milk until well combined.

Nutritional Information

- It is rich in potassium, calcium, and healthy fats.

Serving Size: 1 smoothie

Preparation Time: 5 minutes

5. Strawberry Kiwi Cooler

Ingredients

- Strawberries

- Kiwi

- Greek yogurt

- Coconut water

Preparation

- Blend strawberries, kiwi, Greek yogurt, and coconut water until smooth.

Nutritional Information

- High in vitamin C, calcium, and probiotics.

Serving Size: 1 smoothie

Preparation Time: 5 minutes

6. Pineapple Mint Refresh

Ingredients

- Pineapple chunks

- Fresh mint leaves

- Cucumber

- Lime juice

- Water

Preparation

- Blend pineapple, mint, cucumber, lime juice, and water until refreshing.

Nutritional Information

- Rich in vitamin K, vitamin C, and hydration.

Serving Size: 1 smoothie

Preparation Time: 6 minutes

7. Chocolate-Banana Protein Smoothie:

- **Ingredients**

    - Banana

    - Chocolate protein powder

    - Almond milk

    - Flaxseeds

- **Preparation**

    - Blend banana, chocolate protein powder, flaxseeds, and almond milk until creamy.

- **Nutritional Information**

    - Protein-packed with added calcium and omega-3s.

- **Serving Size:** 1 smoothie

- **Preparation Time:** 5 minutes

8. Tropical Turmeric Smoothie

Ingredients

- Pineapple chunks

- Mango

- Turmeric powder

- Coconut milk

Preparation

- Blend pineapple, mango, turmeric powder, and coconut milk until smooth.

Nutritional Information

- Anti-inflammatory properties, high in calcium and vitamin D.

Serving Size: 1 smoothie

Preparation Time: 7 minutes

9. Blueberry Spinach Power Smoothie

Ingredients

- Blueberries

- Spinach leaves

- Greek yogurt

- Chia seeds

- Water or almond milk

Preparation

- Blend blueberries, spinach, Greek yogurt, chia seeds, and liquid until well combined.

Nutritional Information

- High in antioxidants, calcium, and fiber.

Serving Size: 1 smoothie

Preparation Time: 6 minutes

10. Coconut Banana Dream

Ingredients

- Banana
- Coconut water
- Unsweetened shredded coconut
- Ice cubes

Preparation

- Blend banana, coconut water, shredded coconut, and ice cubes until smooth.

Nutritional Information

- Hydrating and rich in potassium and electrolytes.

Serving Size:1 smoothie

Preparation Time:5 minutes

CHAPTER 6

7 days meal plan

Day 1

- **Breakfast:** Greek Yogurt with Berries and Almonds

- **Lunch:** Salmon and Quinoa Salad

- **Dinner:** Grilled Salmon with Lemon-Dill Sauce

- **Snack:** Yogurt and Berry Parfait

Day 2

- **Breakfast:** Spinach and Feta Omelet

- **Lunch:** Vegetable Stir-Fry with Tofu

- **Dinner:** Vegetarian Spinach and Chickpea Curry

- **Snack:** Cheese and Whole Grain Crackers

Day 3

- **Breakfast:** Quinoa Breakfast Bowl

- **Lunch:** Chicken and Spinach Whole Wheat Wrap

- **Dinner:** Baked Chicken with Sweet Potato Mash

- **Snack:** Carrot and Hummus Dip

Day 4

- **Breakfast:** Whole Grain Pancakes with Nut Butter

- **Lunch:** Mushroom and Spinach Quiche

- **Dinner:** Vegetable and Quinoa Stuffed Bell Peppers

- **Snack:** Trail Mix with Nuts and Seeds

Day 5

- **Breakfast:** Berry Blast Smoothie

- **Lunch:** Salad Niçoise with Grilled Tuna

- **Dinner:** Turkey and Vegetable Stir-Fry

- **Snack:** Cottage Cheese with Pineapple

Day 6

- **Breakfast:** Avocado Toast with Smoked Salmon

- **Lunch:** Quinoa and Chickpea Salad

- **Dinner:** Grilled Vegetable and Tofu Kebabs

- **Snack:** Greek Yogurt and Almond Butter Dip

Day 7

- **Breakfast:** Chia Seed Pudding with Mango

- **Lunch:** Sweet Potato and Kale Buddha Bowl

- **Dinner:** Salmon and Asparagus Foil Packets

- **Snack:** Kale Chips

CHAPTER 7

CONCLUSION

Osteoporosis Diet Cookbook for Women Over 60 is more than just a meal collection; it's a celebration of resilience, a symphony of flavors harmonizing with the body's yearning for strength and vigor.

Each dish has been a brushstroke on the canvas of a better, more vibrant life as you've investigated the origins, symptoms, remedies, and preventive actions. Every dish is a testament to the significant impact of conscious eating on bone health, from the crisp pages of the breakfast chapter to the delicious tapestry of the dinner selections.

This book is a beacon of light in the world of osteoporosis, where the shadows of vulnerability may linger. It's a guide, a friend, and a source of inspiration for adopting a lifestyle that not only manages but overcomes osteoporosis. The path to greater bone health is more than simply a medical requirement; it's an opportunity to savor life with gusto, to appreciate the beauty of each ingredient, and to nourish the body that has carried you through every chapter of your narrative.

Remember, this is not the end of the voyage, but rather the beginning of another. Every meal is an opportunity to reaffirm your commitment to health, to enjoy the delight of culinary creation, and to luxuriate in the knowledge that you have control over your health.

May the flavors remain on your tongue and the wisdom echo in your bones. Here's to a future full of vigor, vitality, and the pure pleasure of relishing every moment. Cheers to you and the exciting chapters ahead!